How To Quit Eating Junk Food

Quickly, Painlessly And Permanently!

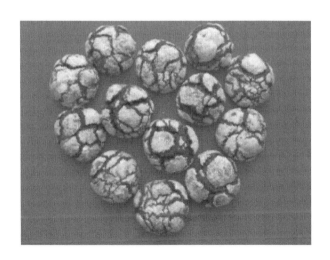

Published By Shaharm Publications

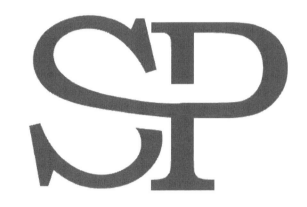

SHAHARM PUBLICATIONS

For a full list of books by Shaharm Publications, please go to:

http://www.shaharmpublications.com

Table of Contents

1. Identifying Your Junk Food Problem

One of the factors that often allows individuals who are addicted to drugs and alcohol to get beyond their addiction is admitting the fact that they have a problem. They may have been addicted to the substance for years, and it may be such a large part of their life that being without it is almost like cutting off an arm or a leg. What many people don't recognize, however, is that junk food is a very addictive problem as well. In fact, there are some experts who believe that certain types of chemicals that are included in many of the junk foods that we consume are actually more addictive than drugs such as heroin and cocaine.

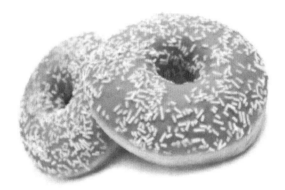

If you are interested in kicking the junk food habit and getting off these types of foods once and for all, this book is the perfect solution for you. Through its pages, you will learn how to identify the problems that you have, and to recognize the solutions that are available to assist you in kicking the junk food habit once and for all. When doing so, it can be a real feeling of freedom and relief, especially when you understand what junk food is doing to your body as well as to your mind.

Junk food comes in a wide variety of styles and sizes. You have sugary junk foods, such as candy bars and jellybeans, but you also have salty junk food, such as pretzels. You have junk food that doesn't really fit into any type of description, such as those that are produced by companies like Hostess and Little Debbie's. These types of foods contain sugar but they contain such a wide variety of other, often unknown, ingredients that it can be quite frightening when you truly know what is inside of them.

Another type of junk food that people often overlook is diet food. Most people feel that if they give up sugary soda in favor of diet soda, they are doing a great service to their body. The fact the matter is, however, the chemicals that are found in diet soda and other diet foods are often so dangerous that they rival or even surpass the dangers that are associated with the junk food that they are trying to mimic. Not only that, many of the so-called "diet" foods actually contain chemicals which are thought to be designed to make you fat. Isn't that ironic?

Discovering What Junk Food Is Doing to You

In the pages of this publication, you will learn what junk food is doing to you, and the type of effect that it is having on both your body and your mind. This information can be quite eye-opening, and it is likely that you will never look at junk food the same way again. Once you are able to recognize that junk food is nothing more than an addictive substance, you'll see the sanity in giving it up, and also the struggle that you may have in doing so.

I'm not telling you about the dangers of junk food in order to make you feel guilty. After all, guilt is a major part of many of our junk food habits, and once we find that we have eaten an entire box of cookies while staring at the clock on the microwave, it is likely that we are having thoughts of guilt. "How in the world did I eat all of those cookies?" or "What is wrong with me?" These are some of the more common questions that are asked by those of us who struggle with junk food addiction. In reality, nothing is wrong with you, there is, however, something fundamentally wrong with a system that allows this type of food to exist in the first place.

Is There a Solution to Junk Food Addiction?

In order for you to truly understand your junk food addiction, it is necessary for you to understand addiction in general. In a chapter that is soon to follow in this publication the subject of addiction will be reviewed in great detail. You will see that it is not only something that is in your head, it is actually a chemical process that is in your brain. When you eat junk food, if satisfies an urge, and as a result, you "learn" that you must have junk food in order to receive the same level of satisfaction.

There are also many psychological reasons why we may be addicted to junk food as well. As you will learn in the chapter on addiction, this is not by chance. The junk food companies have gone to great lengths to keep you in their grips and to ensure that you are not only addicted to their food, you continue to crave more and more of it as you eat it.

If you find yourself in this situation, you certainly are not alone. Many millions of people suffer from junk food addiction, and whether they want to recognize it or not, it is a problem that is having a negative impact on their health. Fortunately, there are things that can be done to help you to break free from the habit and to remain free from it for the rest of your life.

We will discuss a few of the solutions that are open to you, but we also express the need to maintain junk food avoidance. After all, junk food is an addiction, and like all addictive substances, it has a lifelong hold on you. Just one bite of a Twinkie or a single scoop of ice cream could end up sending you in a downward spiral, and before you know it, you're back on the carbohydrate wagon and dealing with all the problems that are associated with it.

We don't need anyone to tell us that junk food is problem. We recognize the fact that it makes it difficult for us to maintain our weight, and it can sap us of our energy, leaving us feeling lethargic and unable to concentrate. If you have found yourself in this situation, take heart. There is help to overcome the addiction, and it is found in this book. When you apply it in your life, you will not only be able to break free from junk food, you will also discover all that life has to offer when you are on the other side.

2. Why Do We Love Junk Food?

In the United States, as well as in many other countries around the world, we seem to have a love affair with sugary sweets and salty junk food. It doesn't matter if you are talking about eating a box of snack cakes or a bag of chips, it is something that seems to have a grip on us that is next to impossible to break. Most people consider this to be a problem with personal morals, or a lack of willpower that causes them to be caught in this cycle. The fact of the matter is, however, it is out of our control.

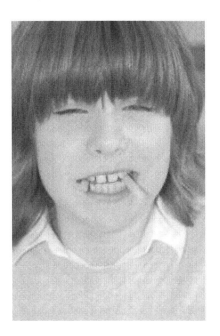

First of all, junk food contains addictive substances, and as such, it causes us to be addicted to it. As you'll see in the following chapter, addiction is a very real issue and it is one that can affect the chemicals in your brain to ensure that you continue to use the addictive substance for the rest of your life. In fact, it even can put you in a downward spiral so that as you continue to foster the addiction, you build up a tolerance to it and continue to eat more and more of the junk food.

Of course, the junk food companies are not complaining about this, because the more of their food that you eat, the more money they are going to make. It is important for you to understand that reality, because it can truly open your eyes to the reasons why you are so addicted to junk food. It is not a matter of personal preference, or even a lack of moral character that is causing the difficulty. It is the fact that the junk food companies go to great lengths to ensure that you are addicted.

Although most people don't realize it, the junk food companies do spend an extreme amount of money to ensure that their food is perfect for you and will cause the addiction to grow stronger. When you understand the tricks that they are using, it doesn't make it easier for you to break free from the addiction but you can begin to see the benefits of doing so. We will discuss how both the feel of the food and the taste of it does make a large difference in how much of that you eat.

Salivation - Our bodies have been pre-programmed to associate the presence of saliva with eating food. Food is something that is necessary for the preservation of human life, and as such, it involves the pleasure centers of the brain and the release of dopamine (more about that in the chapter on addiction). Junk food is designed to make you salivate, and in doing so, it generates pleasure and also increases the taste of the food.

Sensory Input - When you consume junk food, you are eating a food that has a high level of flavor. This is sometimes referred to as flavor overload, and it can reduce the sensation of flavor that you are experiencing. As we continue to eat junk food, our bodies become accustomed to the taste, and eventually, we need to reach out for more taste so that we can enjoy the same benefits as before. Eventually, we eat more junk food, either of the same type or of a variety of types, and fill the pockets of the junk food companies in the process.

Vanishing Calories - Many of the foods that we eat that are in the category of junk food do not stick around very long once we put them in our mouths. This is not by chance, it is by design. When we put a potato chip into our mouths and get that crunch but then the chip quickly disappears, it plays tricks on our brain. Rather than getting full because we are eating excessive calories, our brain thinks that we are not getting enough calories so we continue to eat more and more of the junk food.

Contrasting - Many of the more popular junk foods have a contrast of both flavor and sensation. When this occurs, the food becomes truly addictive. For example, have you ever enjoyed a bag of chocolate covered pretzels? Many people who are junk food addicts find them to be amazing, because they provide you with the sweetness of chocolate, the saltiness of pretzels, and the crunch of pretzels. They also provide something soft for you to bite into that has a crunchy inside.

Turning Off the Safety Signals - One other way that junk food plays tricks on your brain is by providing you with calories but not allowing you to get full. There is a perfect balance of calories within the junk food which will allow you to continue eating it, but it will not allow you to have the satiated feeling that you would get from eating regular food. Have you ever noticed that all candy bars seem to have the exact same amount of calories? The same is also true for many other types of junk foods. This is a design which tricks your body into shutting off the signals that would otherwise be sent to your brain to tell you that it is time to stop eating.

As you are likely now well aware, the junk food companies do not have your best interests in mind. They may produce foods that are taste intensive, but they are only interested in their profits and they will make those profits at your expense or at the expense of anyone else who is willing to use their product. In the next chapter, we will discuss how junk food addiction affects your brain chemicals, which proves to be a truly eye-opening experience.

3. Junk Food Addiction Is All in Your Head

When you struggle to get off junk food, it is more than simply enjoying it and not wanting to give up the enjoyment that you have. In reality, junk food is nothing more than drug food and it affects our brains in much the same way as other drugs, including nicotine, cocaine, and heroin. When you understand the reason why you are addicted and how it is affecting your brain in such a way, it makes the decision to give up junk food easier.

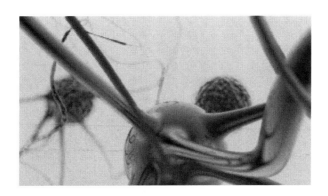

Before we begin to discuss the way that junk food affects your brain, it's important to understand the nature of addiction. Addiction is not a sign of moral weakness, nor is it a lack of willpower. It is defined as a mental illness and one that is irreversible in nature. When you are addicted to a substance, regardless of whether it is nicotine, alcohol, or sugar, it is an addiction for life. You may be able to abstain from the addictive substance, but once you go down that path again, you are helplessly hooked in no time.

The Reward Center of the Brain

There is an area of your brain that is known as the reward center. When you do something that brings you pleasure, regardless of whether it is eating a good meal, drinking water when you are thirsty, or even having sexual relations, it is the reward center that causes you to feel good about it. In reality, it is not just this part of the brain, but it is a complex chemical reaction that takes place as that part of the brain is flooded with a neurotransmitter known as dopamine.

Neurotransmitters, sometimes referred to as brain chemicals, are the chemical messengers of the brain. Your brain cells (neurons) must communicate with each other across the space between the brain cells, known as synapses. It does so by sending these chemical messengers, which are produced within the neuron and passed to another neuron, where they connect through a receptor port. There are thousands of different types of brain chemicals, each which has its own particular function. Dopamine, which is one of the many brain chemicals associated with addiction, is responsible for providing you pleasure among other things.

Of course, the fact that you are getting pleasure from taking part in an addictive substance is more than simply enjoying it. Dopamine has the ability to train you, which is why you crave food when you are hungry or water when you are thirsty. It is a lack of dopamine and a desire to feel that stimulating rush of dopamine on the pleasure center of the brain which keeps you alive. Unfortunately, when you eat junk food, it turns the entire system on its head.

Many Addictive Substances in Junk Food

When you look at the side of a junk food box or bag, you will see an extensive ingredient list. This is only a partial list in many cases of the actual ingredients that are included within the food. Most of these ingredients are there for more than one reason. Although they may have a special "purpose", such as preserving the food or adding taste, they may also be addictive as well. One of the most powerfully addictive substances in junk food, however, is sugar, and we will focus our attention on that drug.

When sugar is consumed, it has an effect on our brain and causes our neurons to be overactive. As a result, there are massive amounts of dopamine that are dumped into the reward center. From the very first time that we consume an excessive amount of sugar, we are beginning the addiction process. It does not take our mind long to recognize the fact that we feel good when we eat sugar, and as a result, we continue to eat it when it is available.

Sugar not only causes the release of dopamine, it also affects the neurons in another way as well. This is through a process known as down regulation, and as we continue to consume sugar, the receptors that accept dopamine begin to disappear. This means that, although the dopamine is still being released in excessive amounts, it is not able to find a suitable "port" where it can attach to a neuron. As a result, we have additional free dopamine in the brain, but it is not having the same pleasurable effect as it had before.

In order for us to continue to experience the pleasure that sugar once brought to us, it is necessary for us to continue to consume more and more of it. This continues to accelerate the process of down regulation, leading to a greater addiction. The entire process of needing to consume more of an addictive substance is something that is known as tolerance. It is likely that you have read about this issue in alcoholics or users of other strong drugs, but the exact same process takes part in sugar addiction as well.

A Very Powerful Addiction

Most people don't make the connection between the addiction to sugar and the addiction to other drugs. If you are addicted to junk food, it is likely that you are an addict, just as somebody who has an addiction to heroin or cocaine is. Yes, sugar is legal and it is included in many different foods, but that doesn't mean that it is any less potent than those other drugs.

You need to be cautious when you have a sugar addiction as well. Many people that are trapped in an addictive behavior, whether it is addicted to hard-core drugs or addiction to sugar, are likely to display that behavior with other types of drugs as well. Many people that have a problem with serious addictions and are in rehabilitation centers end up eating junk food, because it triggers the same chemicals in the brain and provides a limited exposure to the same feeling as the hard drugs that they were taking.

As you can clearly see, sugar addiction is all in your head, but it is not a matter of your imagination. You are addicted, not to the food, but to the effect that it has on the brain and the brain chemicals that are being released in mass quantities. It is a lifelong addiction, but it is also something that can be limited if you remove the food from your diet. This book will help you to remove it through methods that will work for you.

4. Sugar – Killing You with Sweetness

In the previous chapter, we discussed the fact that sugar is addictive and how it affects your brain chemicals. Just having that knowledge alone can help motivate you to give up junk food once and for all. In this chapter, we are going to take a closer look at sugar and how it affects not only the brain, but the body as well.

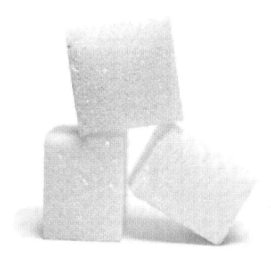

You don't likely need anyone to tell you that sugar is bad for you. When you eat it, it can give you a quick rush, and afterward, will slam you to the ground and make you lethargic, foggy headed, and ready for a nap. Many of us also recognize the fact that sugar is bad for us because of our expanding waistline. In either case, you would be correct to assume that this is a problem with sugar, but why does the problem exist?

How Sugar Is Killing Us With Obesity

Do you know how much sugar you eat every year? If you average it out across everyone that lives in the United States, and you consider yourself to be an average American, you would consume 156 pounds of sugar every year. The next time you go to the grocery store, pick up a 5 pound bag of sugar and imagine that you are eating 31 of those every year, or approximately one bag every 12 days.

The problem is that obesity is at epidemic levels and it not only affects those in the United States, it affects many people around the world. In fact, the United States does not even hold the title for the most obese individuals per capita, that honor goes to Mexico. When most people think about the combination of sugar and obesity, they simply assume that it has to do with the empty calories that sugar is providing in your diet. As you will soon see, the problem goes much deeper than that.

Any type of carbohydrate that you consume, regardless of whether it is in the form of refined sugar, or if it from broccoli, is going to end up as glucose in the bloodstream. Glucose is the fuel that our body needs to run, unless we are on a low carbohydrate diet, in which case the body burns fat for fuel. The impact of glucose on our bloodstream, however, varies quite widely from one carbohydrate to another. With sugar, the glucose moves quickly into the bloodstream, creating an excess that is difficult for the body to manage. Other types of carbohydrate, however, release their glucose slowly, allowing the body to keep up with the load.

The body is an amazing machine and when we have glucose in our bloodstream from the food that we eat, it releases insulin and other chemicals to help assimilate the glucose so that our body can use it. A molecule of insulin attaches to a molecule of glucose and transports it to a cell, where it is used as fuel. If there is too much glucose in the bloodstream, each sugar molecule that is unable to be assimilated is stored as fat in the body until it is able to be used at a later time. Unfortunately, that time never arrives because we continue to load ourselves with sugar, leading to a vicious cycle of fat storage.

It gets worse, however, as we continue to spike our blood sugar levels on a continual basis. Eventually, our insulin can become immune to the effect of glucose and it is no longer able to handle the sugar that is in our bloodstream. This can become a problem with diabetes, but even before diabetes occurs, the excess glucose in our bloodstream becomes a real problem. In order to compensate, our body releases additional insulin, and additional sugar is stored as fat in the body.

Now that you understand how sugar creates obesity, you also understand what needs to be done to solve the problem. In essence, you need to remove sugar from your diet, or at the very least, limit the amount and types of carbohydrates that you are getting to those that are released slowly. You can determine which carbohydrates suit that purpose by choosing those that are low on the glycemic index.

Why Sugar Makes You Lethargic

If you find that you are getting tired shortly after you eat sugar, you certainly are not alone. Many people feel that it is a product of their imagination and that they would be tired, regardless of whether they ate sugar or not. You might be surprised to learn that there is a measurable factor that causes you to be tired and lethargic when sugar is consumed.

In the previous chapter, we discussed how sugar can cause the body to produce a neurotransmitter known as dopamine in excessive amounts. That is not the only brain chemical that is affected by the sugar drug. In addition to causing your body to release excess dopamine into the pleasure center, it also suppresses the production of orexin, which is a brain chemical that helps to keep you awake. By suppressing that neurotransmitter, it makes you feel suppressed, as if you want to fall asleep.

Interestingly, protein has the opposite effect on orexin, but you're not going to find junk food with high levels of protein. This is not because it is impossible to include protein in junk food; it is because the junk food companies want their food to affect your brain chemicals and to keep you addicted. It is just another way in which they are attempting to control your life, and far too often, they are doing so successfully.

5. Wheat – What is it doing to us?

There are many different types of junk food, and contained inside of those foods, there are many different ingredients. One ingredient that is contained in many types of junk foods, including sugary cakes and pies, is wheat. Is this also an ingredient that can cause us difficulties and keep us addicted? The answer may surprise you.

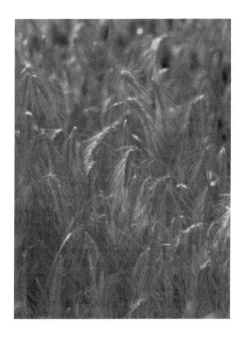

People have been eating wheat for thousands of years, but originally the human race may not have been designed to consume this type of food regularly. At first, we tended to eat a lot of fruits and vegetables and we were hunter gatherers, which meant that we were also consuming a considerable amount of meat as well. At some point within the past few centuries, however, we began to consume more and more wheat products, and it even became a substance that is commonly known as the "staff of life".

The fact of the matter is, however, there may be a lot of problems associated with the consumption of wheat that would make doing so a real issue. First of all, many individuals suffer from wheat sensitivity, either on a minor level that is difficult to detect on the surface, or on a more severe level, such as those who suffer from celiac disease. Wheat that is consumed by somebody who is sensitive to it can lead to issues such as digestive problems, obesity, and brain fog.

It is also interesting to note that the wheat we are consuming today is far different from the wheat that was consumed just a few short decades ago. The modern-day wheat, which is much shorter and produces a higher yield crop, has been designed through genetics and crossbreeding to produce more profit for the growers and for the companies that use the product as an ingredient in their junk food. When most of us envision a field of wheat, we think about tall, flowing wheat plants that are blowing in the breeze. That type of wheat is no longer grown in the United States, but rather, it is a short, stocky plant that has been designed for massive profit.

Wheat may also have a number of other effects on the body that are less than desirable. For example, a condition that is known as gynecomastia, (commonly known as man boobs) may be something that is associated with the consumption of wheat. Gynecomastia is still somewhat of a mystery, but it is thought that the visceral fat that forms breasts on a man may be the result of high blood sugar levels and spikes in insulin levels as well. These are very common when wheat is consumed.

Other issues may also exist, such as problems with your cardiovascular system, issues with your immune system and skin, and even baldness! Obviously, wheat is a substance that is not fully understood, and if it is understood by those that are consuming it, it is likely that they will want to quit consuming it.

Unfortunately, we also have that pesky issue of addiction. Like sugar and many other addictive drugs, wheat is also an addictive substance, and it is extremely powerful. Have you ever tried to give up eating bread? It is practically impossible; although we will discuss ways that you can give up bread and other junk food in this book. Yes, wheat is an addictive substance, and regardless of what the food companies would like you to believe, it is something that is better avoided.

The Chemical Agents of Wheat

When you suffer from a problem with wheat sensitivity, you are actually suffering from an issue with gluten, which is a type of protein that is contained in the wheat. Gluten is broken down in the body, provided your body is able to break it down, and it becomes even smaller substances, known as immunogenic peptides. These are very small substances, some of which are able to cross through the blood-brain barrier and to affect the chemicals in your brain.

This is where the plot of wheat consumption begins to take an evil twist. Those small particles that are able to enter into the brain do more than simply affect the brain chemicals. They actually change the way that you think and make you crave junk carbohydrates, including many of the junk foods that you may have a difficulty erasing from your life as well. It is a well noted fact that individuals who consume wheat eat an average of 400+ calories more every day than those who do not consume wheat products.

This is only a brief discussion of wheat, and there is much that could be said about the subject. It is a substance that can cause severe difficulties for us and it is a major part of our diet, often found in junk food, and can make us crave more junk food and start an endless cycle of addiction.

When you are able to remove wheat from your diet, you will find that you benefit from doing so very quickly.

6. The Benefits of Quitting Junk Food

Like any addictive substance, there are problems associated with eating junk food that can affect your mental and physical health. These negative impacts on your health are often gradual, but eventually, they can overtake your life and can make you fat, sick, and depressed. Fortunately, many of the issues that are associated with junk food addiction are also reversible. In fact, once you are able to successfully get the junk food monkey off your back, you will find that you are experiencing benefits that are often seen very quickly. This chapter lists some of those benefits that you can enjoy.

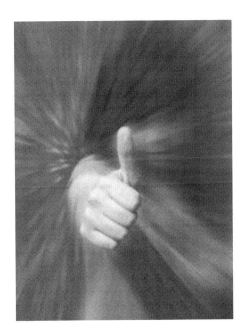

Nutritional Benefits - One of the issues that is associated with junk food is that it does not have any nutritional value. In fact, it is often what could be considered anti-nutrition, in that it actually takes away from the ability of your body to absorb the vitamins and nutrients from any healthy food that you are eating.

There are many different types of junk food that may have this effect on the body. One that is often considered, however, is the fact that wheat causes sensitivities for many individuals, not only those who are known to have celiac disease. It can affect the lining of the digestive tract, through which nutrients are absorbed. As a result of eating the wheat of today, your body is no longer able to absorb those nutrients and you become deficient. This is true, even though you may be eating plenty of healthy foods along with the junk food that you are consuming.

Weight Loss - In a previous chapter, we discussed how the consumption of sugar can cause obesity, and for a fact, is causing obesity for millions of individuals who consume it. Fortunately, the issues that are often associated with sugar consumption are reversible. All that is necessary for you to do is to stop eating sugar and you will begin to recognize the benefits, including weight loss that occur gradually.

Although there are many ways for you to experience weight loss when you cut sugar from your diet, the best way for you to do so is to go on a low carbohydrate diet. This not only removes sugary snack foods from your diet altogether, it also removes other foods from your diet that cause a carbohydrate load in your bloodstream. It causes your body to stop burning glucose for fuel, but rather, to burn fat for fuel, and you lose weight quickly.

Better Physical Health - Many of the chemicals in junk food can lead to health problems, some of which are as serious as strokes, heart attacks, and high blood pressure. These issues tend to creep up on us over time, and at first, we may not recognize that they are a difficulty, but before we know it, we have severe health issues. Most people who eat junk food find that it happened so gradually that they do not notice the connection between junk food and poor health. They end up taking prescription medications which may help to alleviate the symptoms but do not cure the disease.

Better Mental Health - If you have been following the information in this book, you already recognize that junk food can wreak havoc on our brain chemicals. It affects many neurotransmitters, along with having a direct effect on the receptor sites on our brain cells.

The issues associated with your mental health when you are eating junk food can be as severe as depression, anxiety, and stress. You feel a need to continue to consume junk food, not because it makes you feel better on a permanent basis, but because it causes the dopamine rush that makes you feel good temporarily. It is an evil cycle, and once you are in the middle of it, it is difficult to break.

Fortunately, the mental issues that are associated with junk food are often reversible. There may be some damage that is unable to be corrected, but for the most part, you will find that you are feeling much clearer and happier when you overcome junk food addiction than during the time that you were addicted.

These are only a few of the primary benefits that you can experience when you are able to overcome your junk food addiction. More than likely, you will experience some benefits that are specific to you, depending upon your chemical makeup and the type of junk food that you are eating. Continue to enjoy those benefits and to remember the fact that they only happened after you were able to give up junk food.

7. Are You Trying to Lose Weight?

As you have no doubt found through your reading of this publication, there are many reasons why it is a good idea to give up junk food. It can help to correct both physical and mental issues that may have been plaguing us for years due to our addictions to sugar, wheat, and the other chemicals that are found inside of junk food. That being said, many of us were considering giving up junk food, even before we recognized how it affected us on such a deep level. Primarily, this is because many of us would like to lose weight, and we recognize that giving up junk food is a big part of the process.

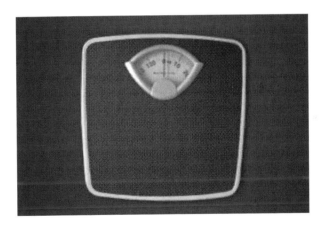

Statistics show that when you are able to remove sugar and wheat from your diet, you are going to lose weight. In fact, many people who remove these two foods from their diet are able to lose 10 or 15 pounds, just in the first week or two alone. This is a significant amount of weight loss, and it can be the catalyst that you need in order to continue with your weight loss efforts.

Many people who want to give up junk food in order to lose weight will not be happy once they reach a plateau. Unfortunately, it can be very difficult to maintain your resolve to give up junk food if you are not seeing the scale move on a continual basis. If you find yourself in this situation, it's important for you not to give into your cravings. At this point, your brain will be trying to trick you and to rationalize the benefits of eating junk food, of which there are actually none.

If you find yourself in a weight loss plateau and you would like to overcome it, there are some ways which work very well in helping to get the numbers on the scale to move again. One of these ways is by eating a very low carbohydrate diet, such as what is recommended on the Atkins diet. This will take some discipline on your part, but you will be surprised with how good you feel and how quickly the scale begins to move again.

The reason why a low carbohydrate diet works so well is because it takes the removal of sugar from your diet to an extreme. Rather than simply removing excess sugar, such as what is included in junk foods, it removes almost all of the carbohydrates that you could consume on a daily basis. As a result, your body no longer has the blood glucose that is necessary to burn for fuel. This may seem like a bad idea, but your body is quickly able to overcome the situation and it begins burning fat for fuel! This can really accelerate your weight loss efforts and can use the fat stores that you may have been carrying for years for its originally intended use, as a source of energy when other energy was not available.

Exercise is also important if you are trying to lose weight. If you have a difficulty with severe obesity and are cutting junk food to lose weight, you should allow the lack of junk food to do its work before any serious exercise routine is considered. You want to make sure that you are not injuring yourself, and if you do exercise, you want to do so within your own, personal limitations.

If you're just trying to drop a few pounds and are not morbidly obese, you can begin to add exercise into your routine immediately. Exercising has many benefits to the body, including improving your mental and physical condition. It can also work along with your dieting efforts, helping you to be healthier and allowing you to shed the pounds more quickly than through dietary changes alone.

You are always going to get advice when you are trying to lose weight. Some of it will be well-meaning advice, while other advice will be from diet companies, which are simply interested in making a profit from your weight loss efforts. You don't need to join a program such as Weight Watchers or Jenny Craig to lose weight. All that is really necessary is to remove sugar and wheat from your diet and you will begin to see the pounds melt away very quickly.

8. Add to Your Diet to Take Away Junk Food

In the previous chapter, we discussed removing junk food from your diet in an effort to lose weight. To be certain, it is the best thing that you can do to help to move the scale in the right direction. The problem is that many individuals suffer from withdrawal symptoms when they attempt to remove junk food from their diet, and as a result, they quickly return to their addiction again.

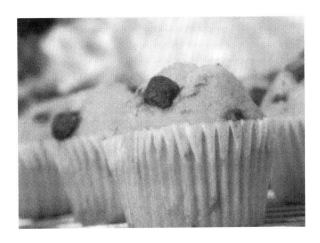

One of the reasons why some people have a difficulty removing junk food from their diet is because they try to make drastic changes in their diet by taking away the majority of the food that they eat. They may rationalize that they are able to benefit because they can remove the junk food while at the same time, replacing it with healthier foods, such as apples, salads, and carrot sticks. In most cases, however, this is a flawed theory.

When you remove food from your diet, regardless of whether it is good for you or not, you are going to go through a period of deprivation. When removing an addictive substance from your body suddenly, including sugar, you will find that the withdrawal symptoms can, at times, be severe. Not only may you experience mood swings and irritability, you could end up with a migraine, or at the very least, a severe headache, because your body is trying to force you to use the drug (sugar) again.

There is also an issue with tapering off food, something that many people try to do when removing junk food from their diet as well. Like all addictive substances, we develop a certain tolerance to junk food, and it is necessary for us to eat a particular amount to enjoy the rush of dopamine in the brain. If you begin to cut back on the amount of junk food that you are eating, you are simply prolonging the agony of withdrawal. It also requires a great amount of willpower to continue to abstain from an addictive substance partially when you are still consuming it partially.

The solution to the problem that you are experiencing is neither to remove the food from your diet suddenly, nor to remove it gradually. Rather, it is to add food to your diet that will eventually block out the bad food that you are eating. What type of food should you add your diet? That really depends upon you as an individual, but many people tend to add a considerable amount of fruit to their diet, along with healthy and delicious salads.

An example of how this might be done can be seen in the typical lunch that is eaten at work. You may have a sandwich that you pack for lunch, but you are also going to eat a Snickers bar, and then it's likely you are going to hit the vending machine for some type of snack cake. In essence, you ate a lunch that is primarily junk food, including multiple sources of sugar and wheat. The only thing that may have been good in your lunch is the lunchmeat, although it probably contained a considerable amount of nitrates. This also is a type of lunch that will never fill you.

In order for you to change the tide, you need to add things to the food that you are eating and to make them healthy. For example, before you eat your sandwich, you could eat a healthy salad, perhaps one that contains some turkey, chicken, or hard-boiled eggs. This gives you a source of healthy, low glycemic carbohydrates along with a source of healthy protein, which will help to fill you. After you eat the salad, you can eat your sandwich, and by that time, you may be full enough that you will not need the Snickers bar or snack cake.

As you continue to change your dietary habits, you can see that junk food is no longer as large a part of your life.

Of course, in essence, you are cutting down on your junk food, but you are doing so in reverse, which is typically accepted better by the mind then trying to cut down on the junk food without providing your body with an additional source of food.

This is just one of the ways that you can change your diet to lose weight without having to suffer as deeply through withdrawal symptoms. Additional lifestyle solutions will be discussed in Chapter 10 of this book.

9. Pulling the Trigger on Carbs

One of the issues that is associated with almost all forms of addiction is the presence of triggers, which make it more likely for you to continue the addictive behavior. This is something that is often seen in individuals who smoke cigarettes, as they will likely have specific triggers which cause them to smoke on a consistent basis. In a smoker, the trigger may be anything from drinking a cup of coffee to talking on the telephone, but it is something that will almost invariably cause them to light up a cigarette. If they avoid lighting up a cigarette during the time that the triggering event exists, their brain will let them know in the form of discomfort.

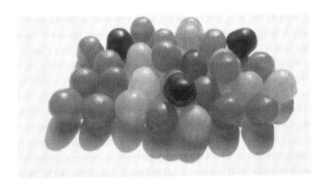

When you are dealing with junk food addiction, the effect can also be measured, just as it can with nicotine or cocaine addiction. There are also many triggers which may make it more likely for you to consume carbohydrates in the form of junk foods, and at times, to do so in mass quantities. In many cases, you may not even recognize the fact that there is a triggering event, and before you know it, you have eaten an entire bag of potato chips or an entire box of cookies, and are left feeling as if you are weak and worthless.

Identifying Your Junk Food Triggers

One of the best things that you can do to help identify your junk food triggers is to keep a junk food diary. For a period of two weeks to a month, you should carry this diary with you at all times, and any time you have a craving for junk food, regardless of whether you fill that craving or not, you should write down information about your day. Consider everything about the moment that led up to the craving, from the specific events that may have taken place, to the way that you are feeling. It is not possible to include too much information, because all of it will be valuable when trying to diagnose your triggers.

It is also important to consider the type of food that you ate when the triggering event occurred. At times, you may have an unusual craving for something sweet, such as a chocolate bar, or perhaps some hard candy. At other times, however, the craving may be for something salty. These cravings differ, mainly because of the effect that these junk foods have on the body. Remember, this is not a random incident, but rather, it is something that is well thought out, tested, and designed by the junk food companies.

Avoidance of Food Triggers

Once you are able to successfully identify your junk food triggers, you need to do something which will help you to overcome the problem. In some cases, this may be avoiding some of the triggers which could cause you to eat junk food. For example, if you tend to eat a lot of potato chips while you are watching TV in the evening, what would be the best thing for you to do? It isn't to get rid of the potato chips, but rather, to stop watching TV in the evenings. The same is also true for any other trigger, regardless of whether it is stress, or your 2 o'clock routine visit to the vending machine.

At times, it may not be possible for you to avoid the triggering event that could lead to junk food consumption. In some cases, this may be due to the event taking place at work and you can't quit your job in order to quit junk food. In other cases, however, it may simply be that you are not willing to change the event because it would cramp your style. If that is the case, you have the option to alter the event to the extent where it will not trigger the desire for carbohydrate junk food consumption.

One way that this could work is seen in the earlier example of eating potato chips while you are watching TV.

Many people consider this to be classic couch potato behavior, but it is destructive behavior, nonetheless. If you assume the same position, laying on the couch with a bag of potato chips on your stomach, eating one after another until they are gone, what could you change about the situation? First of all, you could sit in a chair to watch TV rather than lounging on the couch. You might even try watching TV in a different room, such as the bedroom. In either case, it could be enough to disrupt the trigger and keep you from giving in to the junk food addiction.

Finally, do not be surprised if one type of junk food triggers the addiction and a craving for another type of junk food. How many times did you start out eating a cookie, or perhaps a bag of chips, and before you knew it, you were going through all of the cupboards to find every type of junk food that is available? This is also something that is designed by the junk food companies. They want you to go on junk food binges, and they are very successful at getting you to do so. When you continue to eat junk food, it continues to fill their pockets with your hard-earned money.

10. Three Lifestyle Solutions for Junk Food Lovers

In a previous chapter, we considered the method of adding food to your diet to remove junk food from the diet permanently. This is a method that is very effective, but it is one that is often overlooked. In this chapter, we are going to explore a variety of other methods that can be used to help you to overcome junk food addiction. When used properly, either on their own or in conjunction with each other, they can help you to live a life that is free of junk food and all of the problems that are associated with it.

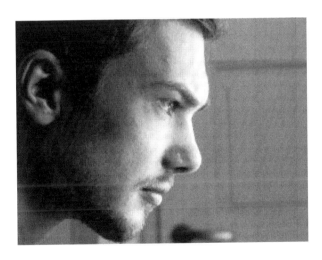

Intermittent Fasting

Another very effective method which can change the way that your body and mind look at the food that you eat is intermittent fasting. This is a method that has been used for centuries, and it has many benefits for both the body and the mind, if you use it properly. Not only can it help you to feel better, it can change the way that your body produces its energy, causing it to begin burning fat for fuel rather than burning sugar. In addition, it can help you to overcome the cravings that are associated with junk food addiction so that it is less of a difficulty to stay free of it for life.

When many people think about fasting, they really have the wrong idea, at least when it comes to intermittent fasting. Intermittent fasting is not about extreme self-denial or living on a mountaintop someplace, drinking nothing but water. Quite simply, it is abstaining from food for brief periods of time, typically for 24 hours or slightly more at a time.

24 hours without food? You might think that this sounds ridiculously difficult but if you do it properly, it is not difficult at all. Rather than going an entire day without eating, from the time that you wake up in the morning until the time that you go to bed, you can do intermittent fasting, while at the same time, eating every day. The real secret is to eat dinner (or lunch) and then to eat the same meal 24 hours later without eating anything in-between. If possible, you can even extend it by eating a lunch one day and waiting until dinner on the second day to eat.

When you practice intermittent fasting, which only needs to be done one to three times per week, it will help to balance many chemicals within the body. This includes insulin, and the way that your body reacts to it. As was discussed in a previous chapter, consuming high sugar junk foods can lead to insulin resistance, which can even turn to type II diabetes, if it continues. Intermittent fasting helps to regulate your insulin levels and to change the way that your body reacts to them.

In order for intermittent fasting to be effective, you need to deplete the glycogen stores in the body. This causes your body to switch the way that it is burning fuel from burning carbohydrates (blood sugar) to burning fat. Since it only takes eight hours for your glycogen stores to be depleted, you could do intermittent fasting every day for only 16 hours. It is relatively easy to do, because you could eat dinner at 8 o'clock in the evening and eat lunch the next day at 12 and that will give you the 16 hour duration that is necessary.

Eating Whole Foods

Another method that many people find to be beneficial is to give up processed food altogether. It doesn't matter if it is junk food or if it is boxed food that is not sugary sweet, it does contain chemicals and is processed in a way that can be very bad for you. Switching to whole foods, such as whole fruits and vegetables can certainly be beneficial for you and will make you healthier, leaner, and happier.

It is also important for you to consider not only the foods that you are eating, but also the fact that you are eating as well. Many of us are afraid of eating fat, because we have been told from a very young age that eating fat makes you fat. Nothing could be further from the truth! As a matter of fact, your body thrives on healthy fats, such as monounsaturated and saturated fats that you get from sources such as olive oil and coconut oil. You may even benefit from eating as much as 85% of your daily calories from these healthy types of fats. This keeps you full, and it certainly can help to curtail your junk food addiction.

Many people try to avoid eating a whole food diet, simply because they consider it to be more expensive than eating fast food or food out of a box. Although there may be cases in which it is more expensive, how much is your health worth? There are also ways for you to cut down on the amount you are spending, including purchasing local foods from a fruit stand rather than purchasing it from a large chain grocery store.

Eat the Paleo Diet

Similar to eating whole foods, as was discussed above, many people find that the Paleo diet fits well into their lifestyle. This diet is high in protein and fats and moderate in carbohydrates. It is often considered to be a low carbohydrate, high-fat (LCHF) diet, and it is one that has many health benefits available with it.

You would be surprised with the diversity that is available when you eat the Paleo diet. Any type of meat can be consumed, and many healthy fats, including real butter, can be a regular part of your diet. Half of your plate will be made up of fruits and vegetables, leaning heavily toward the veggies. It is something that can help you to lose weight, feel better, and to kick the junk food addiction once and for all.

11. Tips to Stop the Junk Food Cycle

Throughout the pages of this book, we have considered many ways to get rid of the junk food addiction and to do so permanently, quickly, and with the fewest withdrawal symptoms possible. In this chapter, we are going to review some of those factors that can help you to get off of the junk food diet and to begin a healthier diet, which will have a positive impact on your life.

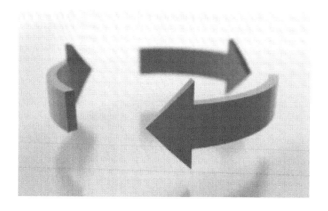

Alcohol Intake - Although a little bit of red wine is healthy and it contains healthy chemicals, too much wine can trigger carbohydrate addictions. This is due to the sugar that is in the wine; although it tends to be a natural sugar in healthier varieties. Another issue with alcohol consumption is that it can lower your inhibitions and make you more likely to give in to your cravings.

Artificial Sweeteners - In an effort to overcome junk food addiction, many people will begin to use artificial sweeteners. They may put these artificial sweeteners in un-sweet tea, or perhaps they may switch from regular Coke to Diet Coke. On the surface, this may seem like a good idea, but in reality, it is one of the worst things that you can do. Artificial sweeteners are chemicals that are known as excitotoxins, and although they may be listed at 0 calories, they affect your brain chemicals, making you crave junk food and keeping you fat.

Water - One of the most important things that you can do for your health and for the reduction of junk food cravings is to drink plenty of water. Most experts will recommend that you drink 8 to 10 cups of water per day, but that may not be enough. According to The Water Cure, it may be necessary for you to drink as much as half of your body weight every day in ounces of water to experience the true benefits that H_2O has to offer.

Plan Your Meals - There is an old saying that if you fail to plan, you should plan to fail. This is a true statement when it comes to any type of addiction, including junk food addiction. You need to plan very carefully so that you don't succumb to the habit again, including packing your lunch for work and making sure that you have a meal plan available through the week. Not only will this help you to have food available so that you don't give in to junk food cravings, it will also help to stabilize your blood sugar levels, which will help you to avoid cravings as well.

No Cheat Day - Many people who would like to overcome junk food addiction do not want to give it up altogether. In an effort to accomplish this, they may be hard on themselves six days out of the week and then for one day every week, the sky is the limit. This may work well for somebody that is not an addict, but if you truly do have a junk food addiction, a cheat day is going to trigger the addictive cycle and you will end up eating junk food continually.

Exercise - The benefits of exercise can never be underestimated. Not only does it help you to maintain a level of health, it also gives you something active to do when a junk food craving strikes. You may be exercising regularly several days a week, but you can also get up and go for a walk when a craving is very strong.

12. Living Free of Junk Food and Loving Life

The information that is provided in this publication can be a very powerful resource, if you use it properly. It has likely introduced you to the fact that junk food, including sugar and wheat, are real addictions. It has also helped you to see how they affect the brain chemicals and even the body to keep you addicted for life.

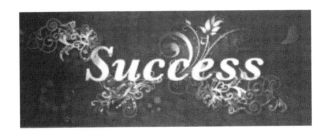

Although it can be difficult to overcome junk food addiction, it certainly is not impossible. When you put the methods that are contained in this book into practice, you will find that you are able to overcome the addiction and to live a life that is free of junk food and all of the problems that go along with it.

Like any type of addictive substance, those that are contained in junk food can get a hold on us and make us a slave to their every whim. Once you are able to overcome the addiction and to gain a level of control, you are not only gaining a level of control over the addiction, you are gaining it over yourself as well.

There are many rewards that go along with stopping the addictive behavior of eating junk food. Those benefits can be felt both mentally and physically, but the personal satisfaction that you will receive is worth every moment that you spend overcoming the addiction. It is a decision that you can make, and once you make it, it is a decision that you can live with.

Made in the USA
Lexington, KY
28 January 2016